THE Girl WHO LOST HER JOY

Until she discovered her superpowers

Written by DPA Weston, PhD

Illustrated by Amanda Shotton

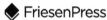

FriesenPress

Suite 300 - 990 Fort St
Victoria, BC, V8V 3K2
Canada

www.friesenpress.com

ISBN
978-1-5255-3932-9 (Hardcover)
978-1-5255-3933-6 (Paperback)
978-1-5255-3934-3 (eBook)

1. HEALTH & FITNESS, CHILDREN'S HEALTH

Distributed to the trade by The Ingram Book Company

Once there was a girl who lost her joy ... until she discovered her superpowers.

Based on a true story, this book highlights a girl's struggle in dealing with a tragic loss in her family. This loss results in the girl developing an anxiety disorder that interferes with her school and home life.

This book shows how all people can learn to deal with challenges from anxiety through persistence, resilience, and a growth mindset.

This book is based on a true story.

This book uses OpenDyslexic
font, an open source font created
to increase readability for
all readers.

Dedication

To MAS: You are missed, every
day, by your family and friends.

M Weston, PhD
2020

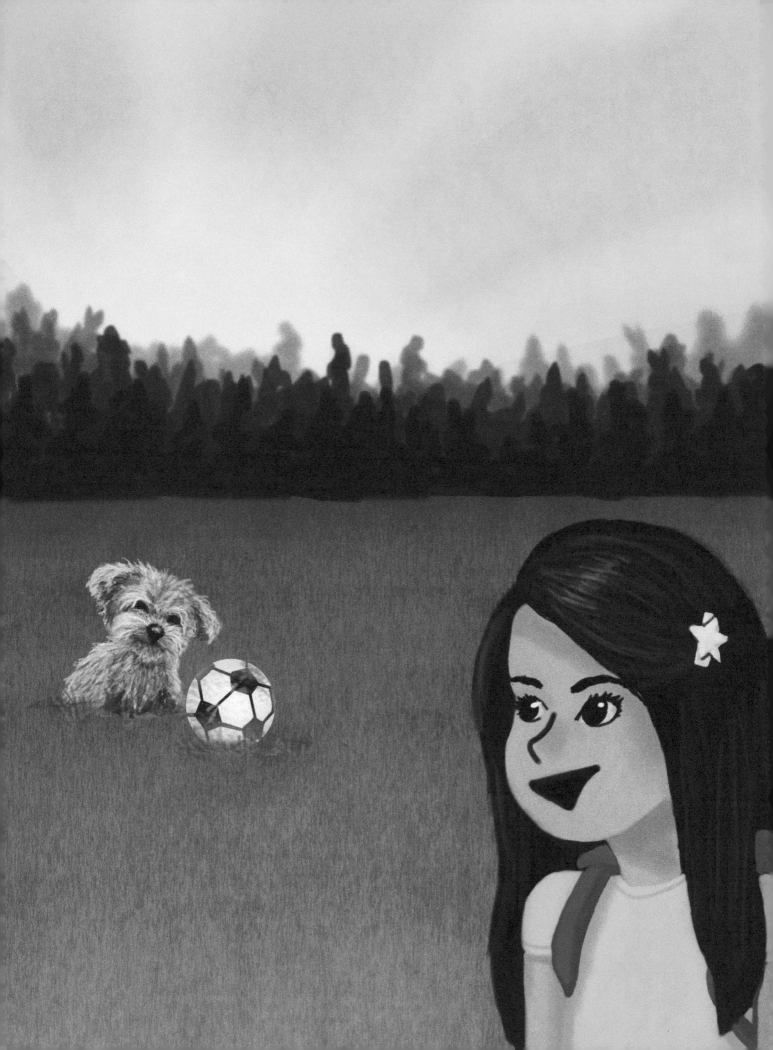

ONCE THERE was a girl whose life was filled with joy.

The girl had a family who loved her very much. She had a mother who lived at one house and a father who lived at another house and an annoying younger brother who lived with her at both houses. The girl had many aunties and uncles and cousins and two grandmas. She had a dog named Oliver who loved to play ball.

Her mother's home was close to the girl's school. Every day, she walked home from school with her friends. The girl played with her friends often. They invited each other over for play dates and sleepovers. It was great fun.

The girl knew she was very lucky to have a life with good food to eat, safe water to drink, a place to feel safe and happy, and people who loved her, including, most of the time, her annoying little brother. It was a good life, and she felt good about herself.

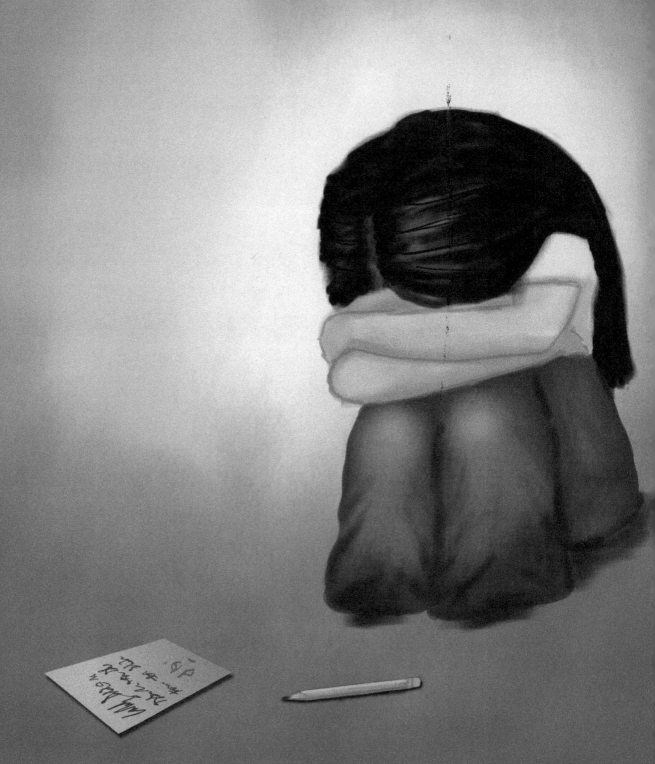

THEN ONE day, a very terrible and sad thing happened.

At first, her parents did not tell her what happened. But when they did, the girl knew she would never see her auntie again.

It was June and the girl was going to middle school in September. Even though the girl had a wonderful summer break, going to camp and playing soccer, she grew sad.

Every day, she grew sadder and sadder. Even Oliver, her dog, could not cheer her up. One day, she became so sad, the girl lost her joy.

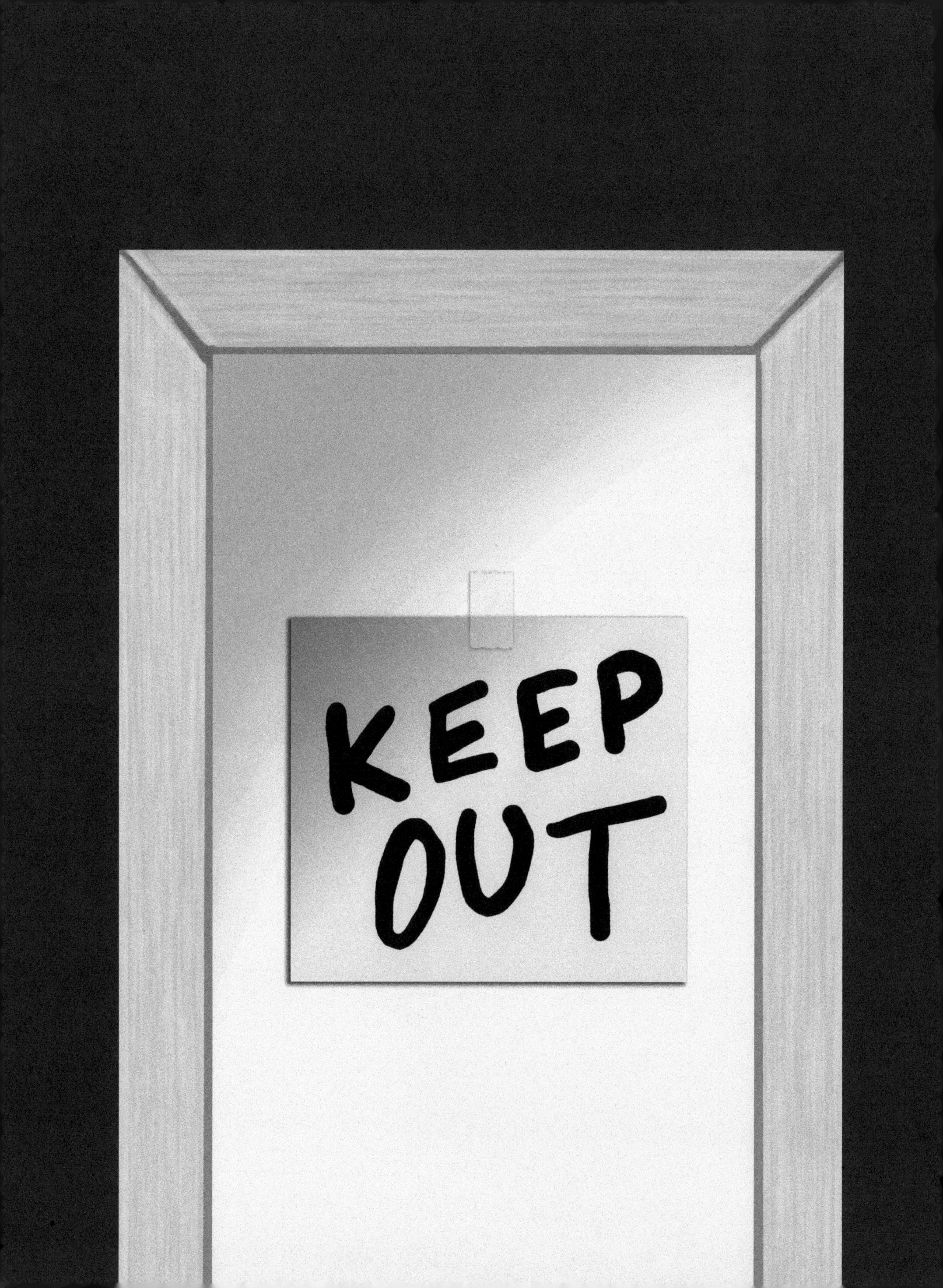
KEEP
OUT

THE GIRL'S mother noticed her daughter growing sadder.

Her mother asked if she wanted to talk with a doctor, but the girl said no.

The girl spent more and more time on her own. She no longer wanted to play with her friends. She spent a lot of time drawing and writing stories in her room by herself.

By the time school started, the girl was very alone.

At school, the girl did not talk to her friends. Her friends were very confused. They came to the house to ask her to hang out but the girl would not talk to them.

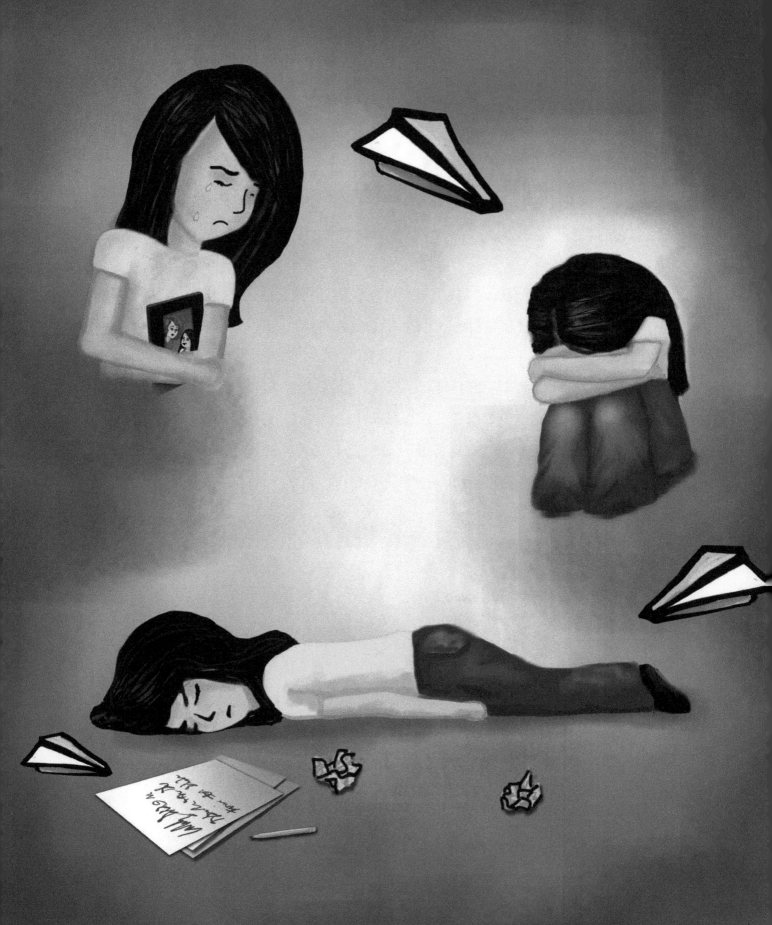

THEN THE girl started having problems. They were not just problems, they were super problems. Some of the girl's problems were that she:

- worried about doing things wrong or being embarrassed
- constantly worried about things she did at school and at home
- had trouble in school either with doing too much school work or no school work at all
- tried to be perfect and worried about making mistakes all the time
- she was afraid to try new things
- had panic attacks where her chest got very tight and she couldn't breathe well
- had many bad dreams and had trouble sleeping
- cried a lot and for a long time
- worried about getting germs, so she constantly washed her hands over and over again until they bled

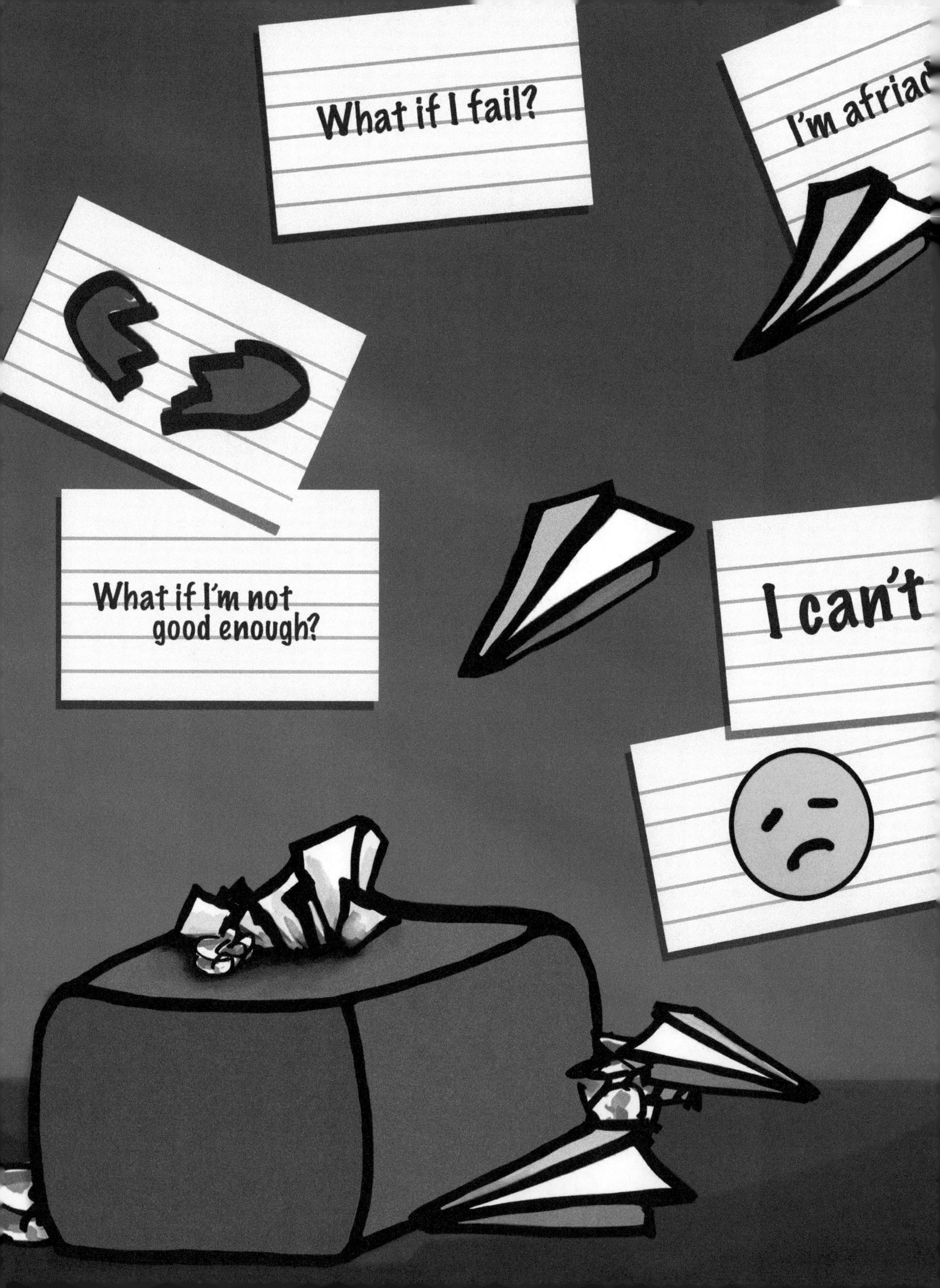
What if I fail?
I'm afriad
What if I'm not good enough?
I can't

THE GIRL'S mother knew something was very wrong. Every day after dinner, the girl followed her mother around the house constantly talking about all the things that bothered her that day.

The girl's parents spoke and decided it was time to get help for their child. They went to see their family doctor. The doctor suggested the girl talk to a youth councillor.

The councillor asked the girl to start writing down all things that bothered her on pieces of paper and then put them in a box. So, she started writing all the things that were bothering her but the box was never big enough.

Every night, the girl spent over an hour telling her mother all the things that worried her. It took a long time for the mother to reassure the girl that everything was all right. After a few weeks, her mother asked the girl to choose the things that bothered her the most and then put them in the box until it was full.

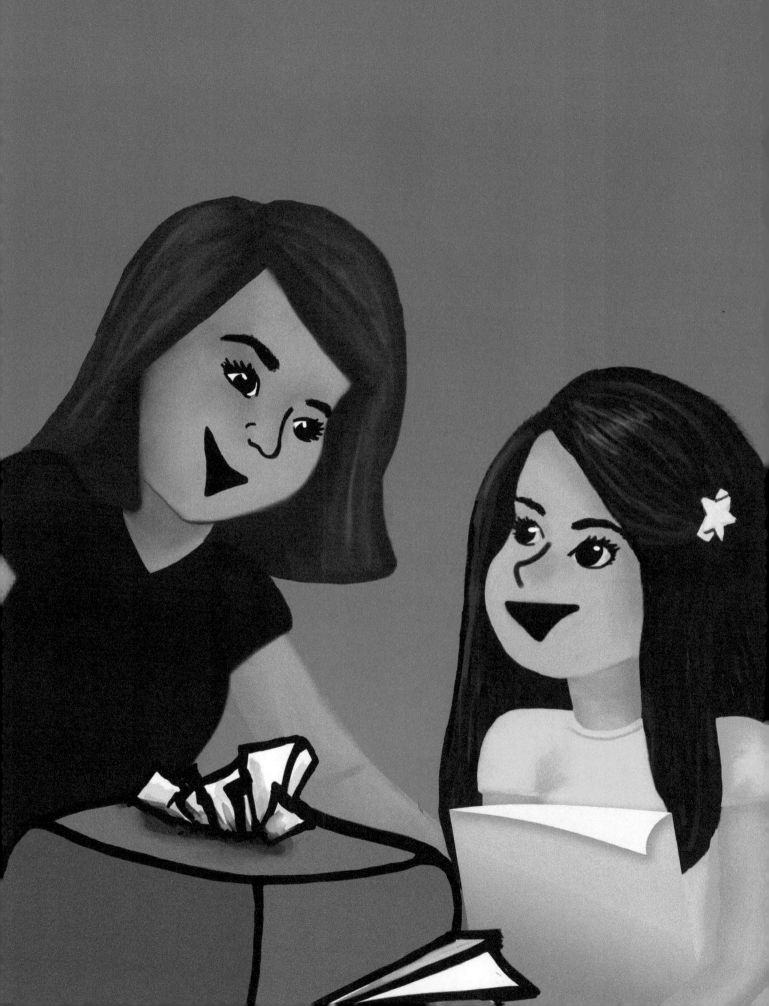

EACH DAY, the girl and her mother spent time together going through all the pieces of paper until they were gone. After a few more weeks, the girl's mother asked her to pick only ten things that bothered her. Each week, the girl had fewer and fewer pieces of paper in her box.

After about a year, the girl felt much better at school. She worked hard in her studies and started volunteering to help others. She worked with other students who cared about the same things she did.

When she finished middle school, the girl's mother thought it would be a good idea for her daughter to have a fresh start in a different school. So the girl went to a new school with kids she did not know and who did not know her. Soon, the girl made many new friends with kids that worked hard at school and were very kind.

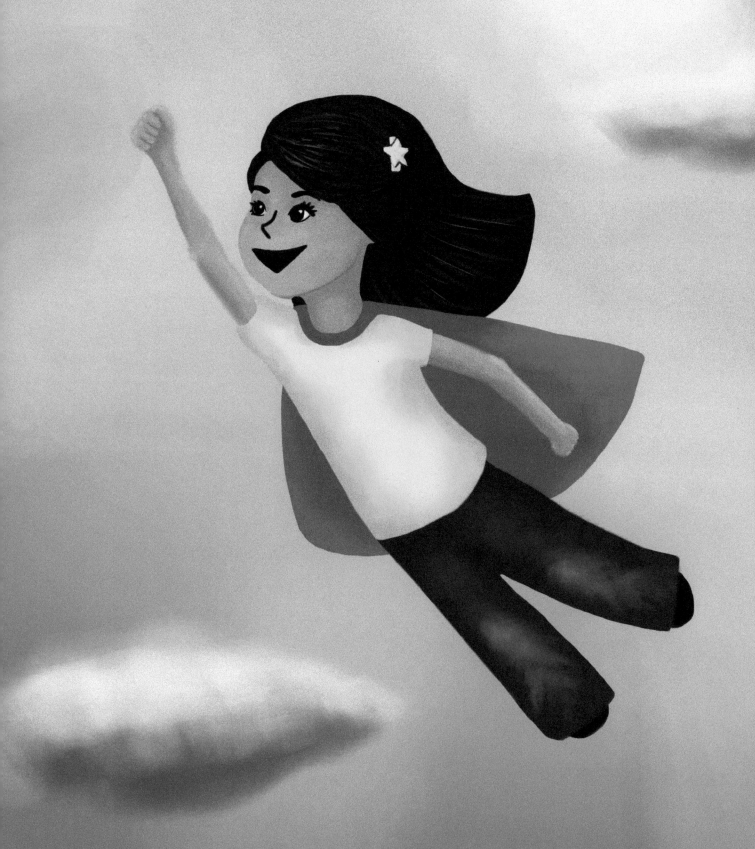

AS THE girl got older, she realized that she was unique, not like other kids in her classes. She started to notice she had super powers that other people did not. Some of her super powers included:

- being highly motivated to get things done
- making lists to make sure she did not forget things
- making good decisions by thinking before she acted
- considering how her behaviour might affect others
- not taking dangerous risks
- being sensitive to other people's feelings
- being intelligent with an excellent memory
- having many interests and always reading
- having a great imagination and loving writing stories
- knowing how to work hard and be prepared for things
- being grateful for her life

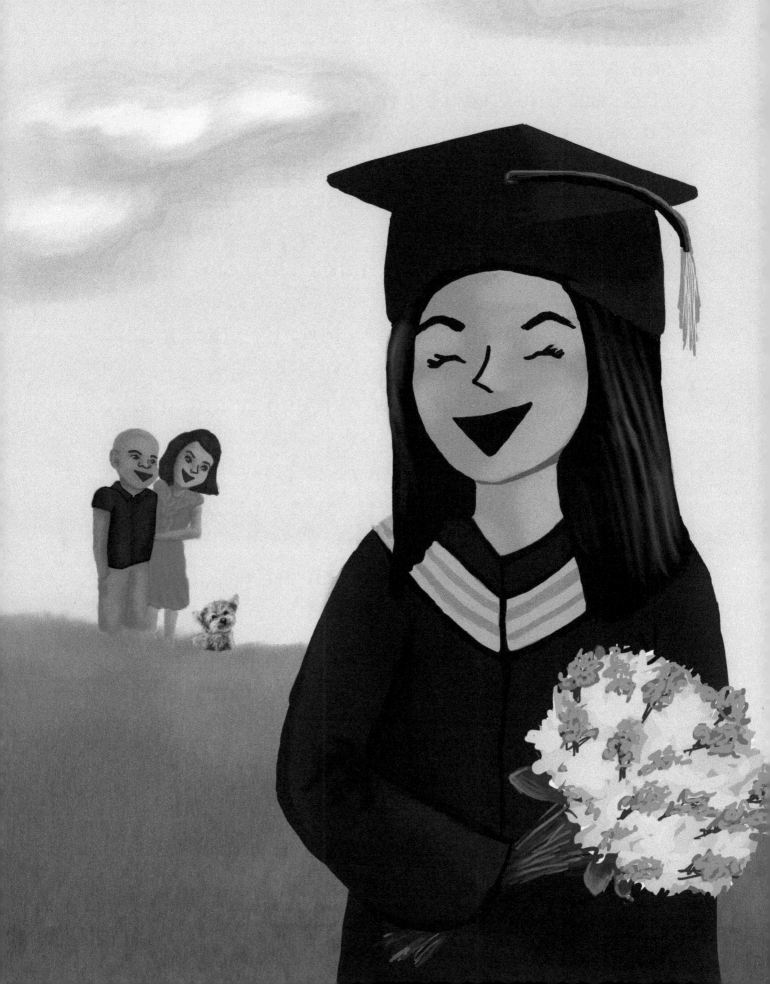

THE GIRL tried new things and took risks.

She started volunteering to help people in her community and in other parts of the world. With her friends, she helped raise enough money to build a school and to dig wells so people in other countries could get an education and have safe water to drink. The girl discovered that she found her joy by helping others.

The girl's health challenges made more sense when the girl's doctor diagnosed her with an anxiety disorder. She found that helping others helped her manage her own feelings.

In her life, the girl learned that she had to keep going when life got tough. She knew that working hard always paid off. The girl grew up to be a talented young woman, went to university and made many new friends.

Today, the girl is still really sensitive to her own feelings and the feelings of others. She also knows that sometimes life can be hard, but with support from friends, family, and community, she can overcome almost anything.

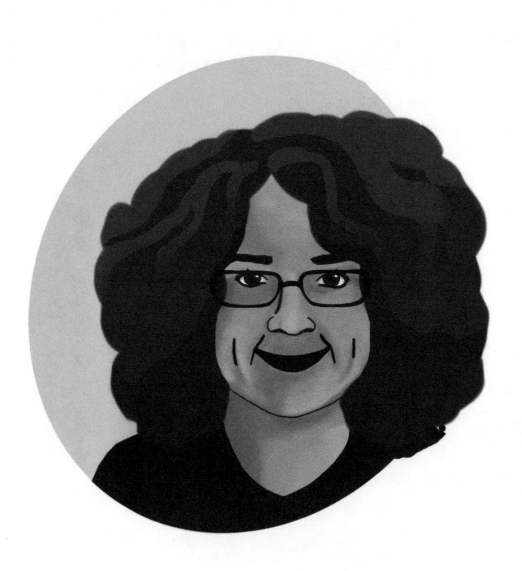

AUTHOR

DPA WESTON, is an elementary teacher who works with students with special education needs in Ontario, Canada. In addition to teaching, Dr. Weston is a writer, instructor, volunteer, and advocate for human rights. DPA Weston loves helping students discover their own super powers.

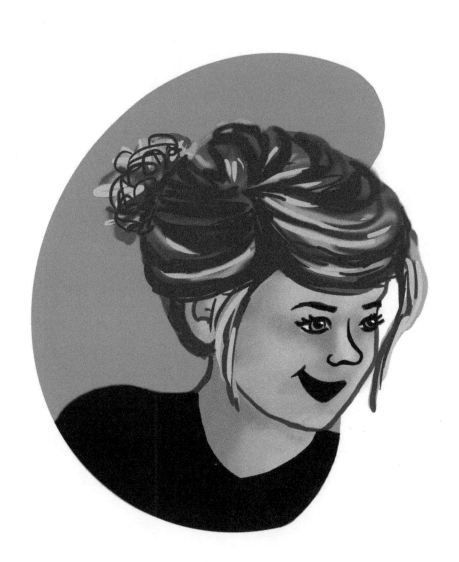

ILLUSTRATOR

AMANDA **SHOTTON,** is an artist with a background in advertising and computer animation who lives in Ontario, Canada. Ms. Shotton loves to show the beauty of life and tell stories with her art.

What's the difference between normal anxiety and anxiety disorder?

Source: Anxiety Canada
https://www.anxietycanada.com/

<u>Normal Anxiety</u>

- Occasional worry about circumstantial events, such as an exam or break-up, that may leave you upset

- Embarrassment or self-consciousness in the face of uncomfortable social situations

- Random case of "nerves" or jitters, dizziness and/or sweating over an important event like an exam or oral presentation

- Realistic fear of a threatening object, place, or situation

- Wanting to be sure that you are healthy and living in a safe, hazard-free environment

- Anxiety, sadness or difficulty sleeping immediately following a traumatic event

<u>Anxiety Disorder</u>

- Constant, chronic and unsubstantiated worry that causes significant distress, disturbs your social life and interferes with classes and work

- Avoidance of common social situations for fear of being judged, embarrassed, or humiliated

- Repeated, random panic attacks or persistent worry/anticipation of another panic attack and feelings of terror or impending doom

- Irrational fear or avoidance of an object, place or situation that poses little or no threat of danger

- Performing uncontrollable, repetitive actions, such as washing your hands repeatedly or checking things over and over

- Ongoing and recurring nightmares, flashbacks or emotional numbing relating to a traumatic event in your life that occurred several months or years ago

How to help a friend with an anxiety disorder?

Source: Anxiety Canada
https://www.anxietycanada.com/

If someone close to you has an anxiety disorder, here are some ways you can help:

- **Learn about the disorder**. Understanding what your friend or roommate is going through will help you give support, as well as keep your worry under control.

- **Realize and accept stressful periods**. Modify your expectations of how your friend should act and be sure to be extra supportive during difficult times.

- Remember **everyone experiences anxiety differently**. Be tolerant, supportive, and non-judgmental.

- **Be encouraging and don't get discouraged**. Give praise for even the smallest accomplishment. Stay positive.

- **Talk to someone**. Being supportive all the time is difficult, so make sure you have someone-a roommate, friend, family member or counsellor-to support you.

Anxiety Disorders Self-test for Friends or Family Members

Source: Anxiety Canada
https://www.anxietycanada.com/

If you suspect a family member may be suffering from an anxiety disorder, print out the test and ask them to answer the questions. Please remember to share the results of this questionnaire with a health care professional.

QUESTIONNAIRE:
HOW CAN I TELL IF IT'S AN ANXIETY DISORDER?

Answer **Yes** or **No** to these questions.

Are you troubled by the following?

- Repeated, unexpected panic attacks during which you suddenly are overcome by intense fear or discomfort for no apparent reason; or the fear of having another panic attack?

- Persistent, inappropriate thoughts, impulses, or images that you can't get out of your mind (such as a preoccupation with germs, worry about the order of things, or aggressive or sexual impulses)?

- Powerful and ongoing fear of social situations involving unfamiliar people?

- Excessive worrying (for at least six months) about a number of events or activities?

- Fearing of places or situations where getting help or escape might be difficult, such as in a crowd or on a bridge?

- Shortness of breath or a racing heart for no apparent reason?

- Persistent and unreasonable fear of an object or situation, such as flying, heights, animals, blood, etc?

- Being unable to travel alone?

- Spending more than one hour a day doing things over and over again (for example, hand washing, checking things, or counting)?

More days than not, do you experience the following?

- Feeling restless?

- Feeling easily tired distracted?

- Feel irritable?

- Having tense muscles or problems sleeping?

- Have you experienced or witnessed a traumatic life-threatening or deadly event or serious injury to yourself or a loved one (for example: military combat, violent crime, or serious car accident)?

- Does your anxiety interfere with your daily life?

Resources:

The **Antidepressant Skills Workbook (ASW)**: gives an overview of depression, explains how depression can be effectively managed according to the best available research and gives a step-by-step guide to changing patterns that trigger depression. (Available in English, French, Punjabi, Chinese, Vietnamese, and Farsi)

http://www.comh.ca/antidepressant-skills/adult/

AnxietyCanada(English): An online patient tools for self-management.

https://www.anxietycanada.com/

Canadian Mental Health Association (English, French): An online tool for self-management.

https://cmha.ca/

MoodFx (English, French): Online and mobile app tracking of symptoms (depression, anxiety, cognition) and functioning.

https://www.moodfx.ca/Resources/

Talk Depression (English, French): Online information, support, and resources related to cognitive symptoms of depression.

http://talkdepression.com/

Daylio (English): An online mobile app to track mood with activities.

https://daylio.webflow.io/

Mindshift (English): An online mobile app designed to help teens and young adults cope with anxiety.

https://www.anxietycanada.com/resources/mindshift-app

Headspace (English): An online mobile app that teaches meditation and mindfulness.

https://www.headspace.com/

What's My M3 (English): An online mobile app for mood tracking.

https://whatsmym3.com/

CPSIA information can be obtained
at www.ICGtesting.com
Printed in the USA
LVHW072147230520
656378LV00002B/16